BECOMING
BIONIC

The Little Book of Hope for Heart Patients

JON KYLE EZELL

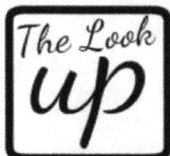

The Look
up
PROJECT

THE LOOK UP PROJECT
57 E. Prescott Street
Columbus, Ohio USA
TheLookUpProject.com
First published in 2011 by The Look Up Project

Library of Congress Control Number: 2011935304
ISBN-13: 978-0615518930
ISBN-10: 0615518931
1. Health / Fitness 2. Healing

Printed in the United States of America
Set in Adobe Caslon Pro Text

Cover design by Gunk Productions
Illustrations by Jon Kyle Ezell

The information in this book is intended to be educational and not intended to diagnose or treat any disease or health disorder. Information contained in this book shall not replace consultation and close supervision with a physician or healthcare professional. The author and publisher are in no way liable for any misuse of the information contained in this book. Readers are responsible for their own healthcare and for making informed decisions that can impact their lives.

becomingbionic.com

Bionic:

Having superhuman
strength or capacity.

This is the book I yearned for during my painful recovery from a heart attack when I was desperate to find hope. A lot of what's in here flies in the face of reason, but hope has nothing to do with reason. I'm not a medical professional, nor do I claim to be. Please visit your doctor and weigh the risks before taking any of my advice.

Why This Book?

I decided to write about my miraculous heart attack recovery story out of concern for all the people who are heart patients. If you are one of them, you might not know what to do other than give up. I almost gave up on hope for my health and for my life, but I decided to find the strength inside of me to fight. You have to decide to do the same thing.

My heart condition changed me forever. I learned that there is a tremendous need to help people "get their minds right," so they can regain their health. I did this. I tapped the healing power of my mind and used it to fix my body. You have to tap yours and put it to work for you. It became clear to me that nobody would be coming to my hospital room or to my home to tell me how to bend my mind so I could thrive again. We're individually responsible for fighting negative thoughts, and it's up to each of us to direct our bodies to respond in the proper way, or we're surely doomed.

This information is also for everyone around you who is not sick. They have no idea how to help you. They love you, but they can't possibly understand the needs of someone who suddenly became very ill unless they've experienced it themselves. They can't comprehend the agony, shock, and mourning that results from losing your good health and the mental and physical impacts that go along with that kind of sorrow. This includes your family, your friends, your healthcare providers, and everyone in your life who has never trembled over The Grim Reaper standing in wait. My story will help them better understand your needs. Pass this along to them after you're finished.

When I needed a voice of hope in my time of crisis I found sympathetic voices, but none could tell me what I am about to share with you in the upcoming pages. It boils down to three things:

1. ultimately, you control your own health and your own future even in the face of adversity (and potentially death); 2. without hope there is no future; and 3. with hope you have a shot.

As your voice of hope, I insist that you devour this material so you can begin the most important work of your life—getting back to good health. Please take a bit of time and read every word right now. By design, it won't take long.

If you are ready, and if you follow through and take command of your future, the words in this book will give you the kind of hope that could bring you a better life than you enjoyed before your heart tragedy. I will be visiting hospitals with several of these books under my arm. I'll also be running around the world to inspire heart patients to take control of their futures. As cliché as this might seem, if I help one person decide to get better, then this emotionally-draining project will have been worth it. And if you purchased this book, I hope you find it to be the best money you have ever spent.

Now, let's get on with my story so you can get on with your fight. *You are about to save your life.*

For My Two Angels

This book is dedicated to two women who helped save my life.

The first is Laura Yamokoski, Heart Failure Team Manager, Clinical & Translational Research Organization at The Ohio State University Medical Center's Division of Cardiology. Thanks a million for choosing me to get those stem cells (or placebo) pumped into my ailing, weak body, and then keeping me laughing and happy for two years during the clinical trial.

This is also dedicated to Laurie Yahl, badass exercise physiologist at The Ohio State University Center for Health and Wellness Cardiac Rehab Center. Laurie, thank you for understanding me and for letting me push boundaries that I was determined to push.

You both are my angels.

You're two big reasons why I'm bionic today.

I'm paying your goodness forward with this project; you've inspired me to want to be an angel to as many people as I can possibly reach.

About the Art

I've spilled my guts in this book, so I figured I might as well share my art here too. I hope you enjoy it.

Fight.

My Story in a Nutshell

At age 41, I suffered a terrible heart attack in my Columbus, Ohio home.

I could have died, and even though I didn't, my heart took a serious blow.

This made me extremely depressed and mad at everyone and everything.

I was lucky enough to be selected to participate in a rare stem cell clinical trial and to receive an intravenous injection of either stem cells or placebo.

I couldn't walk very far, was always dizzy, and had a hell of a time breathing, but the possibility of having stem cells working to build my heart back gave me hope during this desperate time.

Even after a few weeks I still felt miserable. I thought to myself, "I must have the placebo." Hope was sinking like a rock, causing me to fall into a period of severe depression filled with self-pity and thoughts of suicide.

But then I thought, "What if I hadn't been chosen to be in the stem cell trial? What would I have done then?"

I realized that only a few out of millions of heart patients could rely on such a crutch. That's when I decided to kick my heart attack's ass, and proclaimed out loud:

"I am an athlete!"

"I am going to run marathons."

I eliminated fragile hope attributed to stem cells, an as-yet unproven science. My 50/50 shot of having the stem cell injection over placebo was too low. I needed a 100 percent chance of wellness and happiness instead.

Then my heart healed.

I'm better than new.

I feel as if I never had a heart attack in the first place!

Now I have a "bionic heart." I run marathons.

And the big question remains: am I a wonder boy of medical science? Did God cure me? Or is my amazing recovery the product of pure determination?

I'm bionic!

This experience has given me the power and knowledge to spread hope to heart patients who need hope.

If you have had a heart attack or suffer from "heart failure," I am going to teach you how to become bionic too.

My Sour Heart Attack

Nothing hurt.

I didn't complain other than saying to a few people, "Man, my belly feels weird," which evoked an interesting response from a student of mine:

"Well then, woo want me to wub your belly-welly?"

I laughed.

She was right. I had a faint stomach issue. I shouldn't have mentioned it.

Whooptiedoo!

I may have had a runny nose, too. Come to think of it, I also had a paper cut on my pinky finger. It was clear that my little stomach problem was no big deal. But my bout with sour stomach lasted for days.

It didn't get better. It didn't get worse. I chalked it up to finally experiencing my first acute case of heartburn. "Welcome to middle age!"

To soak up the acid I was careful only to eat bland food for days (mostly dry toast), but my stomach condition hadn't changed a bit. No guy can eat dry toast for long. So I decided, "Screw this! I'm having Mexican tonight!"

Wow, did I love Mexican food. I especially loved to use the hot pepper sauce—the hotter the better. Every time I ate Mexican I would pour the hottest habanero sauce I could possibly find over my favorite enchiladas and soft taco platter. My test for good sauce was simple: if the top of my head wasn't soaking wet, then it wasn't worth eating.

I found a particularly sizzling brand of sauce that was clearly meant for a drop-by-drop application, but I poured half of the little bottle on to my huge plate holding a yummy, spicy-hot Mexican platter of (what else?) soft tacos and enchiladas. It felt like heaven when my head bubbled with sweat down onto my face. It also was nice on my stomach because the hotness coated over the sour.

After dinner I went straight home and hit my bed early—full, stuffed, about to explode like a piñata. I was happy.

I remember how I could feel hotness still on my lips even after brushing my teeth.

The next thing I knew I had woken up from a deep sleep—on fire. My clock said 2:05 a.m. My tummy was in agony.

I wished so hard that I could have that annoying sour stomach back because now my stomach was burning out of my body. It was also churning, but I never felt like I needed to vomit. All the while, I didn't see any reason to go to the emergency room for having Mexican food revenge. I would never eat Mexican again! Spending the rest of the wee hours holding my stomach and spitting out drool until 5:00 a.m., I realized that I would probably not get any sleep that night.

As a professor I had to teach a class at 9:30 a.m., and I had already decided that I was going to make it to campus on time. So I jumped in the tub for an early shower to kill a few minutes and find a bit of relief for my stomach by directing my focus onto the comfort of hot water on my skin.

As I moved my head under the faucet to wash the soap off of my face, I noticed something very strange—now my chest felt weird.

It didn't hurt, though; it seemed like it was vibrating manically.

Purposefully, I moved my head under the faucet in exactly the same way, and again I could feel a rumbling inside my chest and a corresponding weird noise inside my head. It was buzzing. I remember thinking it was a sound exactly like the hum of the lightsaber in the Star Wars movies.

Even then, it didn't really hurt, but it was at that moment that I knew what I'd been experiencing had never been just a stomach issue.

Oh my gosh…

This could be a heart attack!

The hospital was just down the street. I was given a bed immediately in the crowded emergency room.

Now I was in excruciating back pain. It was so intense that I followed a strong impulse that called me to kick my legs up and down to keep the pain at bay. I found myself yelling at the top of my lungs, reminiscent of one of those stereotypical baby delivery scenes on television shows.

Nurses would periodically come in. I don't know why, but in their presence I held back my reaction to pain, even while they asked me to look at a "pain level chart." The nurses would ask, "On a scale of 1-10 how much pain are you in right now?"

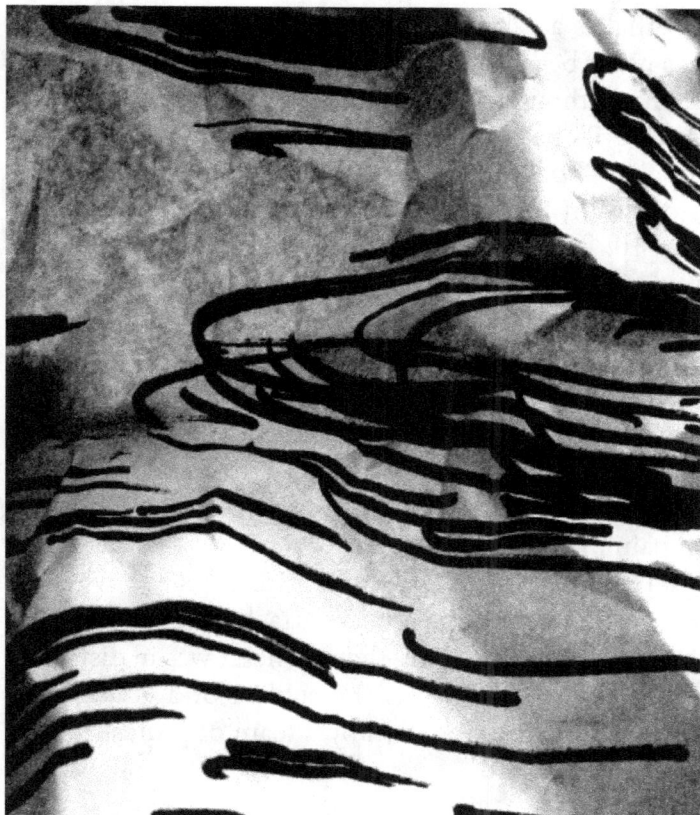

"Pain"

Can you see me in there? Can you see yourself in there?

That is a very strange question for someone who has never been in any significant pain in his life.

Even though I felt like I was a man giving labor to the Devil's baby, for unknown reasons my answer was usually "4" or "6" or some other mid-to-low number. I didn't want to appear dramatic. But soon I was yelling "10!" I didn't care if I appeared dramatic anymore. I was in agony.

I was quickly hooked up to an EKG, and then I was given a shot of something that returned my heart rate to normal, followed by a big shot of morphine.

Suddenly I went from excruciating pain to very little pain at all. I thought to myself how I completely understood why people become addicted to pain meds.

The scurrying ER doctors didn't believe what I was experiencing was a heart attack because my enzymes were not showing that my heart was in distress. At the same time I was the subject of a "Law and Order"-style interrogation by a team of professionals hovering over me:

Them: "Do you do cocaine?"

Me: "No. I've never done drugs of any kind."

Them: "I'll ask you again, DO YOU DO COCAINE?"

Me: "No, I don't do drugs."

Them: "HEROIN? SPEED?"

Me: "I TOLD YOU NO, I DON'T DO DRUGS!"

Them: "It could be your gallbladder."

Me: "But I don't have pain there."

Them: "It could be your aorta rupturing. You fit the profile. Maybe it is your appendix? Maybe it's a phantom pain."

Them: "We're going to wheel you to the CT scan!"

The CT scan results showed that everything was normal, but my attending physician knew something was wrong. I didn't care at this point; I was floating in a pool of morphine and feeling good!

A second blood test taken hours after arriving at the E.R. now showed particular "heart attack enzymes" indicating a heart attack. Yes, YES—*I was having a heart attack!* I was rushed into an emergency heart catheterization session. Now I was on a table surrounded by interns. I could see the doctor in a "DJ booth" in front of me. On my left was a video monitor that would soon display the journey through my body to my heart, so I could watch it happen in real time. Fun! And of course, now I had to pee for the first time all day.

Drugged out of my mind, I put my hand in the air as if that was the signal for "I've got to pee." I grabbed the bedpan off the tray beside my table. Then I was handed a clipboard with a legal form attached. One of the interns said something like, "This says you have a 1 in 2000 chance of dying." That made me confused. How would I legally hold them responsible for my death if I ended up as the 2000th patient?

I signed my life away. I didn't care. I would die otherwise anyway.

The morphine was seriously doing its job by then so I didn't notice the needle inserting the catheter into a big artery in my groin as it readied for the rescue mission to save my heart and my life.

And since I was running on very little sleep during the agonizing night before, this is all I can remember.

Shock and Awe

I was awake in recovery in ICU and I couldn't have been more pissed. How the hell could I, a 41-year old man, have this kind of thing happen to me?

A heart attack? Are you kidding me?

My dad has heart disease, but his first heart attack was at a more acceptable and less embarrassing 55 years old.

A doctor came in to talk to me. "You now have a stent in your ramus artery that was 100% blocked. This was not just a little heart attack. Your heart has suffered some fairly significant damage."

This news made me boiling mad. Perhaps it became damaged during the morning-long wait when the ER doctors were testing my aorta and gall-bladder? How could they not have known that I was having a heart attack sooner?

Then I was shown the results of an important test indicating that my "ejection fraction" (the measure of how well a heart is pumping) had dipped down to near 35% (whereas a normal ejection fraction is around 60-80%). Mine was now half of normal! This test result might not mean anything to you; just understand that 35% is the standard cut-off for heart patients to receive a permanent defibrillator because

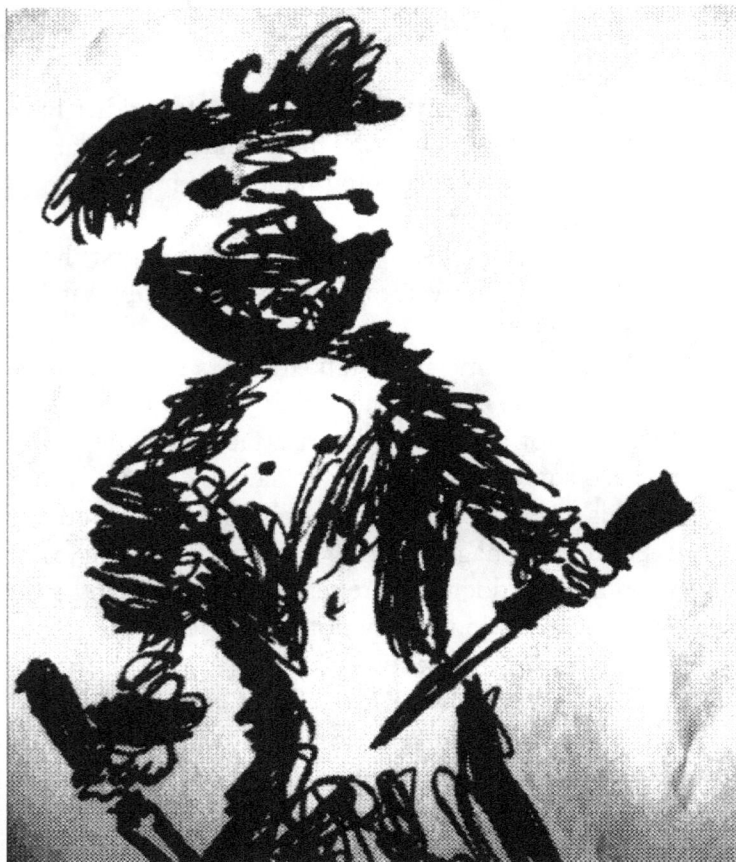

"The Angel of Death"

Curse him! Spit on him!
Then tell him as loud as you can yell,
"I'M NOT READY YET!"

under 35% means a higher risk of sudden death. (As a heart patient you might already know this.)

Sudden.

Death.

Maybe I should have been happy to be alive, but I was mad at God.

I would spit in the Universe's face. I was mad at my body.

I was beyond furious.

There was a lot of chatter by the doctors and nurses using the term "heart failure" (what a terrible, doomsday term that one is!) and what this meant to my future would be shortness of breath, a hard time walking, no running, lots of swelling and, potentially, sudden death.

Great.

Now I was livid.

I was also becoming extremely annoyed by everyone's comments on my age…

New nurse: "Wow, you're too young to have had a heart attack."

Me: "Yes, I know, just gimme the apple juice."

Unfamiliar doctor: "Well then, you're a young one, now aren't you?"

Me: "Yes. Does everyone have to keep saying that?"

New hire test taker: "You're the youngest person I've tested yet."

Me: "Screw off," I thought to myself.

Food deliverer: "Why are *you* in the cardiac unit?"

Me: "Why are *you* trying to feed me greasy meatloaf and mac and cheese the day after I've had a heart attack?"

Food deliverer: "Well, um....."

Me: "You idiot!" I muttered under my breath.

Young-looking garbage collector: "You look like my son's age."

Me: "Go to hell," I whispered not so silently.

This is when I realized that if I emerged alive from hospital hell I couldn't tell anyone about what had happened to me. I would be driven insane. I do not want to walk around having to explain why I am relatively young and had a heart attack. And as a professor, I surely didn't want my students to know what had happened to me. It would crush me to know that my students would now be forced to look at me in a different way, like "you know, that youngish professor who nearly died of a heart attack?" No. Hell no.

In fact, when some students called upon hearing that I was in the hospital, regrettably, I actually lied to them. *I lied to my students!* "No, I didn't have a heart attack, no… no, that's just a rumor."(I'm terribly embarrassed by this. They only wanted to reach out and try to help.) I just couldn't have them look at me as "that dude with the heart attack." I considered myself a vibrant, healthy professor. I couldn't let them down. *No way.*

This was just another good reason to be mad. But now my physical weakness was competing with my anger. And I found out just how feeble I had become when the doctor gave me directions to walk while I was in the hospital.

The nurses took me out in the main hall and stepped off a route where I could walk the halls when I felt like it.

Holding a nurse's arm, I couldn't talk to her and walk at the same time, and I could only go one time around before needing to rest. I felt weird, skipped heartbeats as I walked.

My fingertips felt numb.

My feet hurt.

And I was white hot furious.

Understand that these "laps" from my hospital room to the middle hall were no more than 50 feet. I panted and gasped, deep and loud, sucking for air as if I had been under water for five minutes.

After about three "laps" I was led back to my rollaway bed on the verge of a breakdown and continued thinking, "How the hell could this be happening to me?"

I remember crying as hard as I had ever cried in my life, muffling my sobs, trying to keep anyone from hearing me.

Thank goodness I had a private room.

Next, I became frightened to the point of panic when a nurse brought me a big stack of reading materials. I could see titles that took my remaining breath away.

"Dealing With Heart Failure"

Oh Lord, I have a failed heart. No wonder I can't walk.

"Treating Your CAD"

My what?

What in the world is a CAD?

How on God's green Earth can I possibly treat something I don't know what or where it is?

Is my broken heart a CAD?

"Drugs for Patients Who Suffered a Heart Attack"

You have got to be kidding me.

No, no... now I have a pill regimen—Plavix, Lisinopril, Metoprolol, Eplerenone, Niaspan, Simvastatin, and an adult aspirin. *Seriously? Should I go out and buy a... I can't say it... I can't even think about it... a... PILL BOX?*

Now I would be swallowing a handful of pills that were (gulp!) keeping me alive when just days before I only took a single multivitamin?

Then I started reading the first few sentences of the long list of side effects for one of my new drugs, and it read like watching the most realistic, blood-curdling horror movie ever released, so I declined to read any of the rest of them.

Although I was in the hospital recovering from a heart attack, it didn't take too long to realize that it was my soul that was in trouble. It was quickly turning cold, hard, and dark.

I was beginning to understand that my heart attack was no match for the emotional crisis I was undergoing.

Maybe that's why I didn't have the strength to pray, meditate, or do anything positive for myself. I felt that I was quickly losing the battle of my will, and I knew, deep down in my newly-damaged heart, that I had to get myself together.

It's just that I had no idea how.

This is when my heart attack adventure gets really interesting.

How I Met My First Angel

With my pill materials still on my lap, a nurse knocked on my door asking me if I was interested in being in a clinical trial. I found this odd. I had just had a heart attack, and I was almost immediately asked by a nurse to become her guinea pig. I didn't bother to listen to her and still don't remember the subject of the clinical trial. "No," I said. "No, I don't want to be in any clinical trial. Please ask someone else," I replied as politely as I could.

It wasn't long until another nurse, a very attractive woman with bright eyes and strawberry hair, appeared at my door.

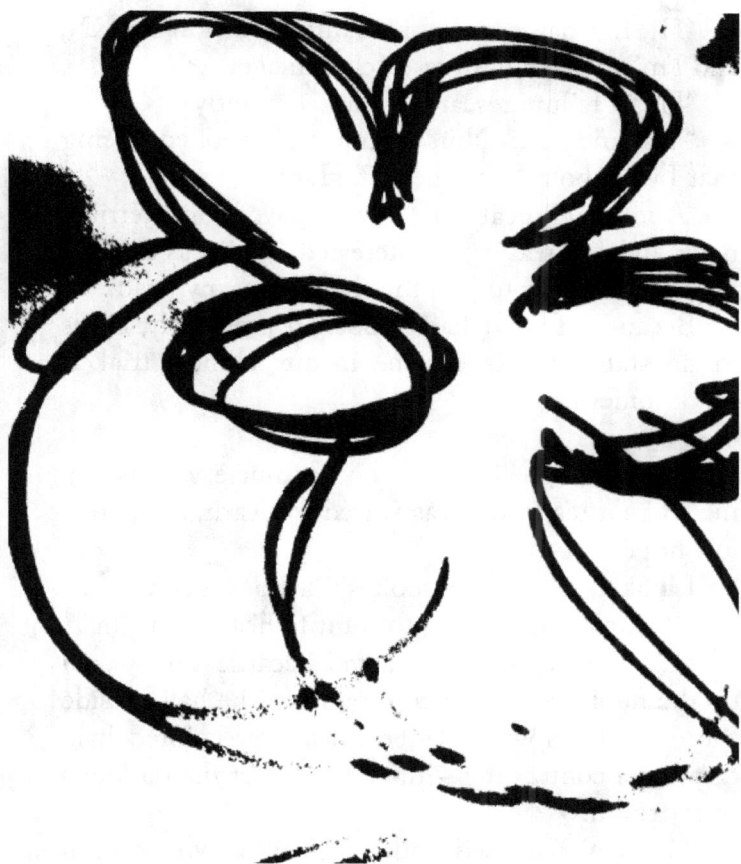

"My Flower Angel"

This is a sketch that represents Laura Yamokoski to me. I will forever be grateful to you.

"Hi, my name is Laura Yamokoski. I'm an RN, and I'm a heart failure research manager...."

"Heart failure research?" I asked quietly.

"Yes, and I...." Nurse Yamokoski replied, seeing that I was about to cut her off. Hard.

"Another clinical trial? I just received some terrible news and I'm really not interested," I said as I rolled my eyes, wanting to pull the sheets over my head.

Because of what had happened previously, I was in no state to help anyone in any clinical trial at that moment.

I was mad.

I was in disbelief that another nurse was asking me to be a test rat. I was scared to death, and I had lost hope.

I looked at Nurse Yamokoski, who was now smiling, "I think you're going to want to hear about this."

She looked like a red angel because she soaked up the fluorescent light coming from the hall outside the door. It showcased her strawberry-colored hair, creating a contrasting silhouette against the darkness of my room.

"Oh yeah?" I asked snidely. "Okay. So what do you have for me?"

"Stem cells," said Nurse Yamokoski.

I pushed the button on my remote control that sat me upright in my rollaway bed. Then I looked at her with wide eyes.

"Talk to me."

My Bag of Stem Cells

I knew about stem cells. They had been all over the news. I knew that they were very controversial. Political fights had been brewing for years about harvesting embryonic stem cells. (Or "dead baby cells," depending on where you are in the debate.)

I remembered reading articles and watching television segments featuring Michael J. Fox, the actor who suffers from Parkinson's disease, and how he lobbied George W. Bush, the president who banned stem cell research during his tenure because he considered their use immoral (i.e., "We shouldn't save adults by killing babies.").

Fox pleaded with the president to allow stem cell research to continue for him and millions of other people who had diseases that might be cured by these cells. I remembered reading about Barack Obama's first day in office and how he made it okay for stem cell research again. Anyway, whatever. I'm not trying to be political. The point is that, as a topic, stem cells are hot enough to have gotten the attention of more than one president.

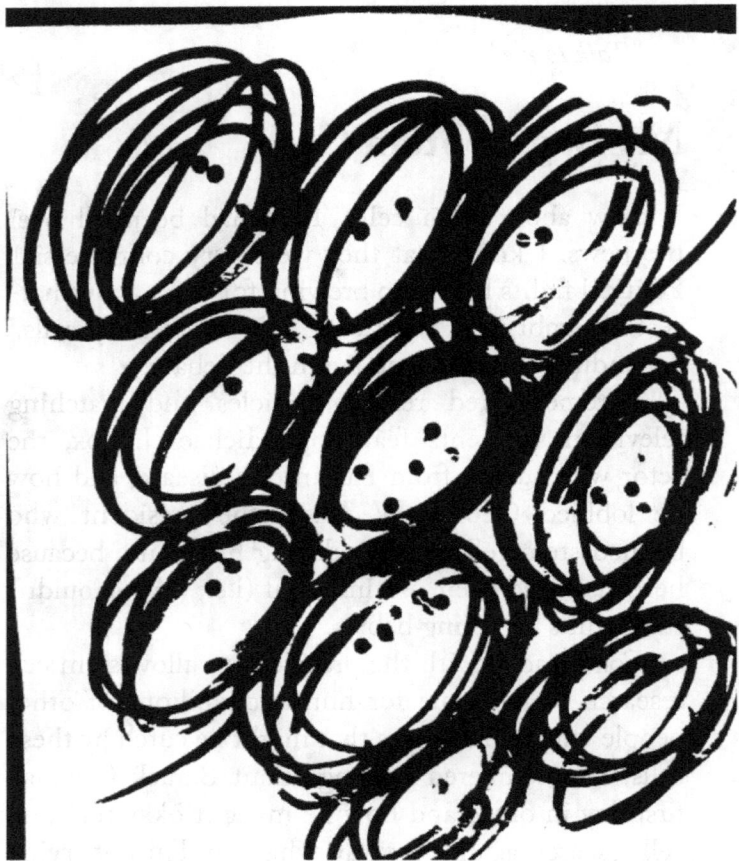

"Stem Cells Waiting"

In the bag, ready to be deployed.
You've got millions of these in YOUR BODY. Deploy them.

I grew up watching Michael J. Fox in the *Back to the Future* movies and on the *Family Ties* sitcom. I respected the fight in him. If he thought stem cells were that important, I was absolutely thrilled to tell Nurse Yamokoski that I was interested and would gladly sign all the documents necessary that would get those little buggers inside my body as soon as possible to repair my weakened, sick heart.

For those of you who may not know how stem cells work, I'll give you the dummy's version as best I understand it:

> Cells are the building blocks of our organs. There are heart cells and liver cells and lung cells and cells that make up every part of our bodies. Stem cells are not yet programmed because they are not a "heart cell" or a "lung cell." Stem cells can form into any kind of cell. They are waiting to morph into some other cell form.

> When our body parts have damage of any kind, they send out chemical signals that say, "I'm in trouble, and I need help."

> Stem cells go straight to where they're needed because they "hear" those chemical

S.O.S. signals. For instance, in my case, I had heart damage, so any stem cells would know to go straight to my heart, take the form of heart cells, and replace and repair the damaged cells, and therefore, create a new heart for me—one that was as if it never suffered tissue damage caused by a heart attack.

Our bodies already have stem cells that do this kind of work. This clinical trial I signed up for involved intravenously pumping millions of extra stem cells (or placebo) from an IV bag directly into my veins, and they would quickly find their way to my sick heart.

So in theory, bombarding bodies with infusions of fresh stem cells could spark a revolution in human regenerative tissue.

Although I was unlucky that my heart was damaged enough to qualify to be in the stem cell trial, I realized that I might have just won the lottery of health. How exciting! Thrilling even! And my stem cells wouldn't even be controversial; they would be taken from adult donors' bone marrow.

I would be required to spend the next two years in an intensive study where I would be given many kinds of tests to see if the stem cells "took" or not.

That sounded good.

No matter what, I'd get a lot more attention than ordinary heart patients would.

Or I would be poisoned like a guinea pig in a mad scientist's laboratory. I didn't care.

Preparing for My Stem Cells

Before I could be cleared to receive the infusion, I'd have to be put through many tests to see if I had anything else wrong with me.

Did I have cancer?

Did I have liver issues?

Kidney issues?

Did I have *any* other disease, big or small, other than heart disease? The answer was no. I passed all tests! So, now that heart disease was absolutely the only ailment that those little stem cells would want to swim toward and try to fix, they (or placebo) could be pumped into me.

It wasn't certain if I would actually get stem cells. As in every blind trial, I would be given either a big bunch of fresh liquid stem cells shot into my veins or

I would receive a big, wet bag of placebo juice. The 50/50 odds seemed like good odds to me.

I felt a strong urge to get ready for my stem cells. I needed to feel some control over influencing the odds. If I shaved and showered and looked somehow "worthy" of stem cells then the technicians who would be setting up the infusion would be more apt to give the real stuff to me. This is preposterous, I know, but it seemed logical at the time.

I pushed myself up, sucked in some air, and slowly stepped into the hospital room's bathroom shower. This time, instead of hearing buzzing in my head and weird things in my chest, I felt what I interpreted to be the power of God and the light of hope covering my body as I washed and shaved. I had been chosen to get an opportunity to live fully again with the help of potent stem cells.

As I washed my body, I was also washing away the trauma and embarrassment of the heart attack.

This shower was spiritually exhilarating, but it was also physically painful because I could barely breathe, I was swollen, and I was tethered to wires. But suddenly I wasn't sad anymore. I had big-time hope. All negative emotions were beginning to quickly evaporate, which was the best gift I could have been given at that time. I was so appreciative of my 50 percent chance of getting 100 percent better. The idea of stem cells made everything bright again.

Amazingly, my outlook had changed on a dime. I had the hope I needed.

Freudian Slips

Clean, shaven, and in a fresh hospital robe, I felt like a kid on Christmas Day.

Nurse Yamokoski stopped by.

"Are you ready for your stem cells?" she asked.

"I'm getting stem cells for sure?" I beamed.

"No, I meant ready for either stem cells or the placebo," Nurse Yamokoski replied.

"Yeah, right!" I teased. "Since you said stem cells I'm sure you *know* I'm getting them."

Nurse Yamokoski smiled and shook her head.

But I knew that I was going to get the stem cells. Perhaps I'd get them because I was a youngish heart attack victim and the team wanted to know how I would respond versus an older survivor? Maybe I would get the cells because the staff knew that I was a professor and that I would be an ideal subject, stay on track, and therefore keep their research in line?

Or, most likely, the staff knew that I was a good guy who deserved another shot at a full, healthy life.

I was going to get them.

A male member of the research team came into my room to tinker with the machines and begin the set up process.

"Are you ready for stem cells?" he asked.

I knew, like Nurse Yamokoski, that he meant stem cells or placebo, but I saw his question as yet another positive sign.

"Yes." I smiled. "Yes I am."

The Hope-Infused Infusion

Nurse Yamokoski and the rest of her stem cell research team began piling up in my hospital room.

A woman in a white hospital scrubs brought in an Igloo cooler. I was thinking, "How sci-fi this is!"

A technician unfolded an IV tube that had an amber-colored plastic cover over its length so nobody could see what was being pumped into me. (I surmised that the placebo would have been clear saline and therefore colorless, but I couldn't know for sure.) Another nurse attached the covered tube to my existing IV needle. Several other staff members were there to watch the procedure. I guessed that they were there to witness the process and to make sure that there were no mistakes in protocol.

I was elated. This was all for me! I was going to be well soon!

Then the woman in the white scrubs opened the Igloo cooler. I tried to get a glimpse of the bag but it was covered with more camouflage. She hooked the bag up, replacing my saline bag.

"Here it comes," said the male technician.

When the liquid made its way through the amber-colored cover it felt ice-cold as it hit my veins. Stem cells needed to be kept cold or they would not survive, right? I took the coldness as another positive sign that I was absorbing actual stem cells and welcomed the pain in my frozen arm.

A pungent sulfur smell filled the room, and I considered this to be another clear indicator that I was getting the real stuff. I surmised that something as powerful as stem cells couldn't smell like flowers.

My future was bright. I was the luckiest man alive. Now I was ready to go back to school to teach!

Hope But No Air

I insisted against the doctors' advice that I would teach my next class just three days away on Tuesday. Teaching was my favorite thing to do in life. I just couldn't lose that! I had to get to class at all costs, even if that meant telling everyone that I felt fine when I clearly didn't.

If you remember, I had already decided that I would keep my heart attack quiet from my students. And, if you recall my concern, other than not wanting pity, I surely didn't want to be driven insane with comments about being too young. (A poor, unfortunate 41-year-old with a heart attack.)

But everything was great in my mind.

All I could think of was that I probably had stem cells.

Hooray, hooray!

I had them.

I just knew that I did.

I arrived early to the building where my classroom met so I could make sure not to see anyone before I could get settled.

This was an undergraduate class, and it was early in the quarter. I was hoping it might be possible that the younger students didn't know my habits well enough to notice any big change.

Unfortunately, I forgot about one of my best students who lived far out in the country and, as a rule, arrived very early so she would have time to study. She approached me at the elevator, asking, "Hey, why aren't you walking up the stairs like you always do?"

Students notice things, and she noticed that I always hoofed the four-story climb, sometimes with her.

I just looked at her.

I didn't have the energy even to respond because it was all I could do to stand without holding on to a wall. It was like being back in the hospital trying to walk my 50-foot "laps" and losing air fast.

I stepped onto the elevator and let the door close. What that student must have thought—first, no response to her question. Then a slow turn away as if I completely rejected her, followed by an awkward step into the elevator, another slow turn back, looking back toward the student in silence as the door closes in her face! This had to be the most bizarre and droll comedic movie scene ever played out in real life!

In the elevator, I sucked in as much air as I could on the way up, white-knuckling the railing, and hoping against hope that my student wouldn't be waiting for me in the opening on the fourth floor.

I began to realize how hard it was going to be to fight off dizziness and what was becoming a constant feeling of doom.

How in the world would I get through the lecture?

How in the hell would I make it through the day?

It took me a long time to get from the elevator to the classroom, about 200 feet away. I'd walk a few feet then lean against a wall for a few minutes. A few more feet, a few more minutes. I'd talk to students as they came in and passed me, surely wondering why I was "reading" with my back resting against the concrete block wall.

Finally, I made it through the classroom door. Now I had no wall to grab and was, by necessity, walking like a crippled penguin. The students were very curious. They knew something was up because I could see their amusement over my tiny steps and ridiculously deep breaths that made my fairly-flat belly fly out from my pants and back in again, and my hands stretched out for anything I could hold on to.

They didn't say anything. Some looked away, which was even worse.

As you can imagine, that lecture was hell on Earth.

I was so dizzy. My sentences were as short as my lung capacity. I did the very best I could, but the students began to whisper and I could almost make out some conversations: "What's up with him today?" I'm sure every student knew that something was up, but coming clean was out of the question. I would somehow have to find a way to do a much better job of faking my condition.

After class it took me 45 minutes to get to my bus stop. It would have ordinarily taken 10 minutes. I spent 15 minutes trying to get out of the building, then 30 minutes to walk across campus to the main street. I will never forget this because it was one of the most surreal trips of my life.

I can remember being on the campus sidewalk and feeling like I was in the Twilight Zone.

Everyone around me was young, obscenely robust, and grotesquely healthy.

I felt like the oldest living man—or should I say— the most nearly-dead human on Earth.

Hundreds of gorgeous, virile, energetic kids kept passing me, three-by-three, then five-by-five, waves of perfection, taunting me, startled by my unusual slowness, wondering what the hell was wrong with me as I shuffle-stepped my way to the bus stop.

But it was all okay. I probably had stem cells. I had hope. Everything would be great.

Only days before I would have been filled with rage during my walk to the bus stop, but as I continued shuffling, I kept telling myself how lucky I was to have a 50/50 chance of having stem cells swimming inside my body, and how they were tinkering with my heart and making me whole again.

My mind was in a place filled with hope and anticipation for good things in the future. I'd soon join the sidewalk kids and blend in better. It would only be a matter of time.

It was on this day that I appreciated just how important having hope is. With hope you have everything. Without hope there is sadness, anger, and potentially death.

I finally made it to the bus stop.

Upset and Anxious

For a month I kept up this "I'm okay" charade.

I was getting good at looking and acting normal in public. But it was hard. Mastering the art of grabbing double breaths and trying to use extra-long sentences so I could finish a thought before the dizziness set in during conversations was exhausting—especially when there were no walls available to lean on or chairs to sit in.

Somehow, and I can't believe I pulled it off, I was able to live a somewhat normal life by faking good health as best I could, and then I'd go back home and fall apart in private.

It was during this time that I had a routine physical checkup that turned my world upside down.

I was being put on a watch to see if I would need surgery to insert a defibrillator.

I had forgotten about how I could experience sudden death—a real possibility for me due to my low heart function. I still refused to call it heart failure.

Without one of these devices attached to my heart and ready to shock it back to life, instead of shuffling, gasping, and grabbing my way to my classroom, I might be lying face down somewhere on campus.

As upsetting as this was, it was starting to make sense. Here I was, still barely able to walk and breathe

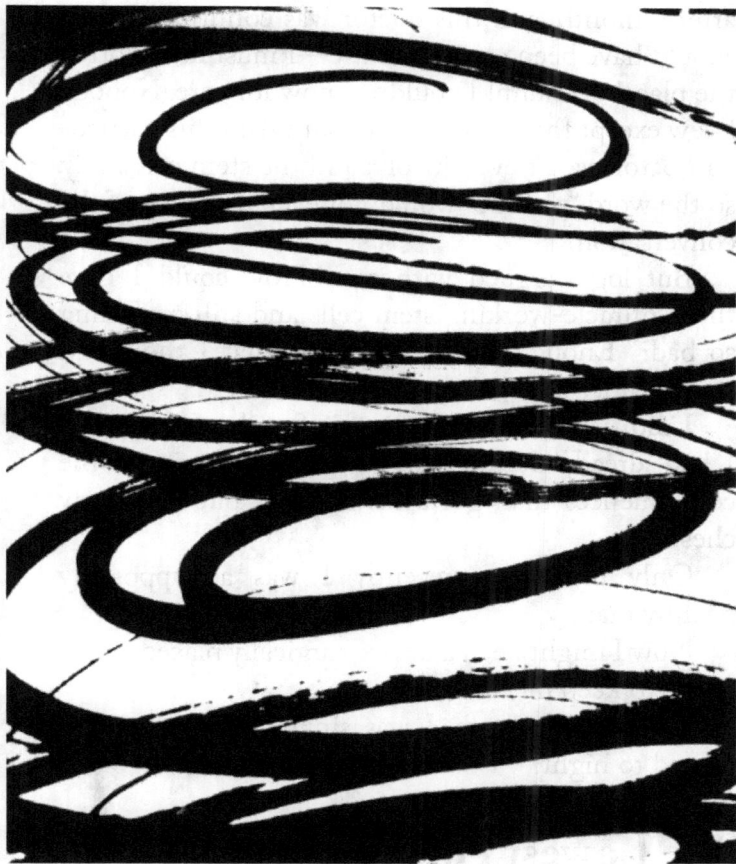

"Dizzy"

Your outlook becomes dizzy when you're worrying and wondering
about your health. Catch your balance now.

after a month, and this doctor was confirming what should have been obvious to me—I must have gotten the placebo. Damn! I couldn't know for sure. Nobody knew except the stem cell company. And this particular doctor wasn't even involved in the stem cell study, so the word "placebo" would not even be a part of the conversation.

But logic argued with me: "How could I have those miracle-working stem cells and still be feeling so bad?" Enough time had passed that I thought I should at least feel okay.

I didn't tell the doctor, but before I left his office I had already decided that I would rather face the consequences than get a defibrillator put inside my chest.

Only until very recently I was a supposedly healthy man.

Now I might need a device surgically placed inside of me to keep me alive?

I was losing hope. I was sinking fast. Then day turned to night.

The Lowest Point of My Life

My unread heart disease reading materials were piled on the floor in my bedroom. A brochure entitled,

"How to Handle Heart Failure" happened to be on top of the pile. I took the brochure and climbed into bed. It should have been a boring read, but it was alarming.

> Major heart failure symptoms:
> Fatigue and weakness? Crap. Check.
> Swelling in your feet? A little bit. Shoot. Check.
> Irregular heartbeat? Uh oh. Check.
> Shortness of breath upon physical exertion? Double check.
> Shortness of breath when using only one pillow when lying down?

Hmmmm. I was lying down, and I felt okay, but I use three pillows and have my whole life, so I threw two of them on the floor. Now, laying nearly flat on my back with only the one pillow, I could barely breathe. The world seemed like it was going dark. I was gasping for air and reaching to the floor to grab up those pillows. Then I turned out the lights and stared up to the ceiling and began whimpering like an abandoned puppy.

Bawling, I choked and coughed so much that I was feeling worse than using only the one pillow, struggling to find oxygen and beginning to wonder why I should even bother.

That night let me know what hell must be like. From what I know, besides the heat and flames, hell is a place where people are desperate and have no hope for anything to get better—ever.

It was clear to me that there was a distinct possibility that, indeed, I might not get better. Maybe I would have taken this easier if I were 99 and had had years to prepare for my death. If I were destined to get worse at such an unacceptable age to die, then I decided that there was no point in life anymore.

Life as a young (albeit middle-aged) invalid could never be in the cards for me. I wouldn't allow it to be.

If a defibrillator machine were put on my heart now, who knows what would be next for me?

It was at that very moment that I decided it might be better if I checked out. I wasn't ready to become the oldest middle-aged man in the Midwest. I would die on my own terms, with dignity!

This was a weird feeling. I really didn't want to die. I had so many things I wanted to do—a million things. And until very recently, I thought I had decades to live. Now I wondered all the time when I would die.

I didn't get the stem cells.

Stem cells would save me.

Instead they're saving someone else.

Life is cruel.

God is mean.

The world sucks.

And I can't bear to live as a functioning invalid faking my way through life for much longer.

This was, without a doubt, the very lowest point of my life.

I continued to cry.

I cried for the person I had become and mourned my good health as if I were at my own funeral. Although I didn't know how I would put an end to my life, or even if I could go through with it at all, I could easily see myself dead. It was okay. I would be better off. After all, hope was gone.

Good feelings were gone.

So I could easily be gone, too.

I contemplated suicide for what seemed like hours in my dark bed.

I Saw the Light

After I had cried myself out, I turned on the television. A documentary on Holocaust survivors popped up on the tube.

These brave people were talking about how hope had kept them alive even as the smell of burning flesh hovered in the air—the burning flesh of their friends and family. They talked about how hope gave them the strength to believe that tomorrow would be a better day and that happiness was on its way. Hope kept their minds from breaking down and hope kept their emotional spirits intact, so they could plan their escape.

I was embarrassed.

My little heart failure problem seemed like a joke. I still had a life because I was alive.

Wait, I thought. What if Nurse Yamokoski hadn't have come into my room? What would I have done if (like everyone else in the world) I hadn't received the possibility of stem cells? Would I still feel as sorry for myself as I did at this moment?

Would I have downed a poison martini by now?

Without the stem cell injection, where in the world would my hope come from?

I AM ALIVE!

I could have been one of the quarter of unlucky people who drop dead during their heart attacks.

Then I thought about my doctor. He is only trying to help me. He wants to help keep me alive by putting a high-tech defibrillator in my body that, maybe, after a while, I would forget about if I could somehow learn to walk and breathe again.

"Poor me," I said out loud in the most sarcastic way possible. Then, there are the millions of people who didn't get to live even half of the interesting, great life that I had been fortunate enough to live—even if it was only 41 years.

Other than my currently shaky health status, I had a lot going for me.

All I needed to do was to get better.

I just had to get better. I decided that I had to ignore the fact that I could have received stem cells.

I couldn't rely on science alone. I had to rely on myself. I decided that the best way to achieve a new reliance on myself was to give myself a goal.

I needed to find a goal that would propel me into health. It had to be a goal that was inspirational to me and simple to understand with clear measures and outcomes. I thought to myself, *"I want to be the complete opposite of who I am right now."*

"Who am I now?" I asked myself.

Well, I was sickly, out of breath, and couldn't walk without dizziness or wall-holding and slow shuffling. I was pitiful. I did not want pity from anyone. I thought about what kind of person was the very opposite of sickly and pitiful.

Hmmmm....

Wait....

It was quickly becoming clear to me what kind of person I would decide to become.

I pushed myself into the bathroom, flipped the light on, put my head to the mirror, looked directly in my eyes and shouted at the top of my lungs:

"I am an athlete."
"I am a runner."

I had run in the past but mostly on treadmills in the gym, and I played basketball in high school, but I never considered myself an athlete.

I was just an average Joe.

I loved the idea of becoming a real athlete and a real runner.

Runners don't gasp for air, and they don't have to hold onto anything when they stand.

Runners have magnificent bodies.

They look healthy and vibrant.

They're competitive and unafraid.

So "runner" was absolutely the opposite extreme descriptor for what I currently was. And it made me happy to think of myself in this way. But not only would I declare that I was an athlete, and, in particular, a runner, I had even bigger plans for myself:

"I am going to run a marathon."

I smiled at myself, and myself was smiling back at me. Now I was on track. Who cares if I only received the placebo?

I am still going to be magnificent.

My Outlandish Rehab

I joined cardiac rehab at the Ohio State Medical Center's Center for Wellness and Prevention a few weeks after I had decided that I would become an athlete. Though I was weak as water, I was already a runner and a seasoned athlete in my mind even before I arrived at rehab.

I was assigned to Laurie Yahl, my awesome trainer/exercise physiologist and my second angel.

Laurie competed in figure competitions all over the United States. She was also a runner.

A runner!

Laurie was magnificent.

She was the picture-perfect image of health: tight muscles, confident posture, and glowing personality.

She could help me get to my marathon. But I actually told her that I was interested in doing a half marathon.

I didn't want to scare her.

But as a goal, running a half was just as scary as running a full marathon for someone starting cardiac rehab less than two months after suffering a devastating heart attack.

After my first day at rehab, Laurie might have been thinking, "Yeah, right, you nearly fell off the stationary bike after a minute. And you think you're going to run 13.1 miles?"

But she wasn't.

She could see and feel my determination. She knew I meant what I said when I said I wanted to be a runner.

It's amazing. When someone means what they say, even against incredible odds, other people seem to automatically want to help you reach your goals. Positive thinkers attract positive people.

Besides, outlandish goals are fun to try to achieve—like traveling to Mars or finding a cure for cancer. Those are big ideas worth rallying behind.

So is running a long race after suffering a devastating heart attack. *Outlandish!*

So while all of the other patients walked on their treadmills, Laurie put me on a running regimen, very slowly and in tiny intervals at first, but I wasn't allowed to run during the first week. I could barely walk three miles per hour for only a few minutes, but in my mind, I had finished an entire marathon.

In about the third week I began testing running slowly for about 90 seconds, and I was thrilled. During those few seconds I told a story to myself, so I felt like I was actually running a marathon. My mind was ready and my body would follow!

Astonishingly, I was up to a *quarter mile* at *six miles per hour* the very next week! Oh my gosh! A quarter mile! Now only 104.8 more of these to go and I will have completed my first marathon!

(Note: I was under intense supervision and hooked up to an EKG. The cardiac rehab staff was ready to scrape me off the floor. If you had a heart attack, please join cardiac rehab; it an incredible, confidence-building experience!)

With every step, I could see myself running in my marathon. I would pretend that my fellow rehabbers were the crowd cheering me on. As I was running, I continued to have vivid, colorful, inspirational thoughts about the marathon I would be enjoying soon. See if you feel inspired by my running script:

I look fantastic in my lime-green tank top and black shorts as I proceed fast and steady along the course. To spectators it seems as though I'm barely breathing. That's because I'm in such good shape.

And wow! I just can't believe my legs! *A runner's legs.*

They're ultra-slim with long muscles that are perfect for running long distances.

My legs continue magically pumping and pushing even after thousands of repetitive steps, gladly carrying my body forward toward my goal as though it is a robust eight-cylinder engine and my legs are its pistons.

My lungs are clear. My muscles are flexible and strong. And my heart is dependable, flawless, and driving those pistons by efficiently delivering oxygen to my hungry cells.

I'm particularly impressed by my shoulders. They're gallantly holding up my back muscles, those heavy bones, big organs, and pounds of flesh, dangling below them.

As I progress down a hill the sun pops out of a cloud, hitting my shimmering skin and drawing attention to my entire body— *my beautiful body* that's behaving like a well-oiled machine.

And I can feel the sweat running off my face and hands and quickly drip—drip—dripping onto the pavement below, leaving a long, thin trail of my DNA all over the city.

On the side of the street I decide to grab a cup of electrolytes from a volunteer. As I pound down the cool drink it hits my dry throat and thirsty stomach at just the right time, giving me an instant burst of energy that will easily take me several more miles.

Then I watch the world go by in fast motion, but I catch a few glimpses of much younger people watching me. Little wide-eyed kids are mesmerized by what I am doing. So are the teenagers and young adults.

They think I'm badass.

I think so too.

Even more than this, I see myself as a superhero powered by all of the strength and stamina that is channeled into me from faraway suns. I look up to the sky as my way of saying thanks for this magnificent capsule that my soul inhabits, appreciating that it did exactly what I asked it to do for me.

There's the finish line! People are waving at me and cheering for me.

Basking in yet another glorious accomplishment, I take a moment to silently cheer myself too.

I know that I'm amazing because wow! I ran 26.2 miles and I know that this is an accomplishment that only a tiny fraction of the population has the courage and strength to do. And I can't wait to do this again.

At the end of the quarter-mile, I thought about celebrating my outlandish goal of a 26.2-mile finish with my hands in the air, feeling as if I had conquered the world.

Using this powerful script, my quarter mile turned into a mile. It was at this point that I created what I called my "heart puppet." This was actually my hand acting as my heart, and I would pump it, squeezing the blood (the air) as hard as I could, pumping the blood (air), so it would reach all of my organs and cells. To describe how this works in greater detail, imagine pulling your fingers out wide as wide as you can but keeping the shape of a human heart, and then quickly squeezing them back in while imagining your real heart is pumping at the efficiency of a 20-year old athlete's heart.

I put my heart puppet to work pumping during every waking hour (not only on the treadmill at rehab). I would pump it so hard that my fingers cramped.

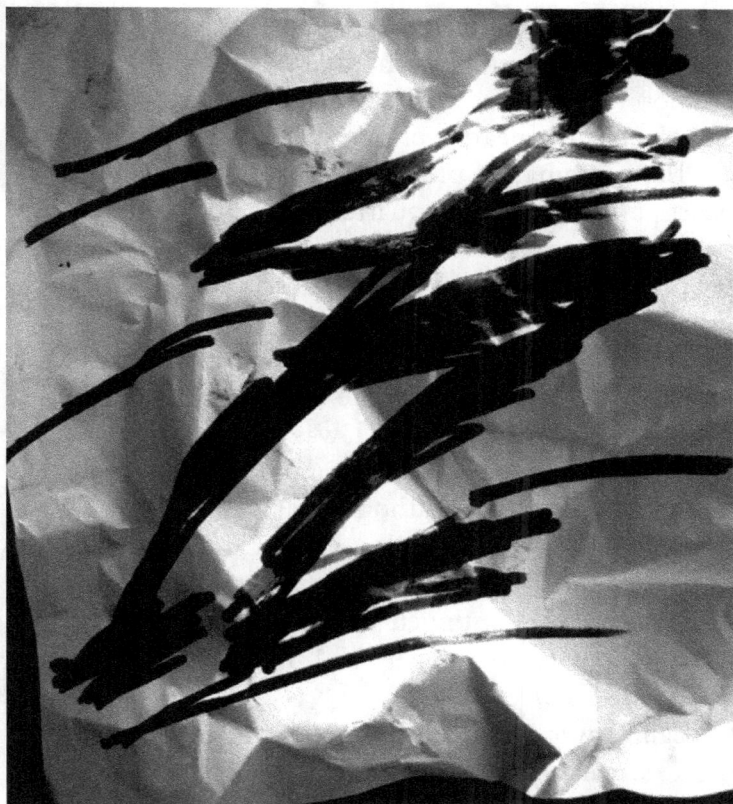

"Me, Runner"

I stare at this piece to reinforce the idea that I am a runner. It's the opposite of who I was—nearly dead, unable to breathe, and hopeless. What do you stare at to remind yourself about who you will be?

But every time I ran, I pumped—and pumped—and pumped—especially hard, imagining that my ejection fraction was normal and robust with an image of a healthy heart ever in my mind.

The combination of my script and employing my heart puppet turned my quarter mile into a mile.

A mile! I could run a mile on the treadmill! Many people who never had a heart attack haven't achieved this level of fitness, but I did!

Hooray!

Cardiac rehab sessions were two hours long, three days a week. I loved them. I was getting better—a lot better. During those two hours the real world did not exist, only the marathon I was running. And I was suddenly logging miles a week, albeit only a few total miles, but miles just the same, like a real runner would. I continued to use my script and my heart puppet. Soon I was up to 1.5, then three miles. *Three mile sessions!*

Laurie was extremely impressed. She was helping to organize a 5K run to raise money for cancer research and told me that she would give her blessing to me to run it. It was only a month away.

That's the very moment when my abstract thought merged into reality. I had become a real runner that day. I could run (the distance of a 5K run) on my treadmill at a respectable speed.

That gave me the hope to go *four miles—five miles—six miles!*

Before the race I could run six miles on the treadmill at a constant six miles per hour. (A steady 10-minute mile.) And to think that this was only several weeks after I was lying in my bed, unable to breathe and thinking about dying.

It was my first race. I would be joining around 300 others. This was a run through a big park in Hilliard, Ohio, a suburb of Columbus. The course was a greenway that used to be a railroad track, and it would take us 1.5 miles out and back.

Several of Laurie's friends were there and many of them were seasoned runners. I seemed to fit in. I didn't feel uncomfortable at all.

I looked like a runner.

I *was* a runner.

Ready... set... GO!

I was running in a real race.

The first time I had ever run off the rehab treadmill.

I played my marathon script in my head, but the reality didn't match. I started in the front of the pack and almost everyone was passing me. But it was okay. I was running. *I was running in a real race.*

Running on the ground is also much different than running on a treadmill, especially when confronting hills. There were several slight hills that nearly did me in. But I didn't care because I was running. *I was alive!*

I started up my heart puppet. I looked down at him as he was sending blood to my legs and feet. He was working hard, and I knew that I couldn't let him down.

As he pumped, I passed the first quarter mile. Laurie was there cheering for me, as were many other members of my beloved cardiac rehab staff.

"Way to go, Jon!" Laurie yelled. I'm sure it must have been truly rewarding for her to see me running in her race after all I had been through. She knew she was responsible for much of my success.

I had crossed the first mile marker, happy. People were still passing me, but I was feeling exhilarated and free.

But then...

A major heart palpitation jolted me.

I had felt this kind of thing in the cardiac rehab sessions, but the staff would tell me that they "didn't see anything" on the EKG and that I was probably okay.

But here I was a mile into a country greenway far from any hospital emergency room and too far from the cardiac rehab staff. My remote location made it impossible to be "scraped up" quickly enough to make any difference.

So I stopped running and began to walk slowly.

"What should I do?" I said out loud to myself.

Then I looked down. My heart puppet was still pumping. I had gotten so used to pumping my hand that it had become second-nature to me. I laughed. Now it seemed funny that I had created a fake heart out of my own fingers. "I must be nuts," I thought. This diversion snapped me back to my script. My palpitation was long gone. I was okay, although I had lost a few minutes, but I would finish this race!

I crossed the finish line in 31 minutes, which was only slightly slower than the speed I usually ran on the treadmill.

The rehab staff was nearly in tears.

We all ate bananas together. I was so happy.

It was one of the best days of my life.

My Super Heart Puppet Hero

My cardiologist ordered another ejection fraction test to see if I needed the permanent defibrillator.

Two days before this test, I decided to create a "super heart puppet" which required both of my hands. I realized that two hands cupped together looked even more like a real heart than one hand ever could. "Frank," my inexplicable name for the super heart puppet, came alive by first cupping my hands together, pulling my right hand out, and then slamming the ball under my right thumb against the ball of my stationary left hand thumb. BANG! BANG! BANG!

The day before my test was not a cardiac rehab day so I decided to go run at my personal gym. I thought that perhaps an extra day of exercise would improve my test score somehow.

Frank and I ran three miles together. Admittedly, it was difficult using both hands to keep Frank going and effectively run, but I did it. And I knew that other people in the gym were staring at me and wondering if I was playing with a full deck. I didn't care. Frank would save me. I kept running, tuned the world out, and visualized my real heart working perfectly.

Flash-forward to the waiting room of the hospital where I would receive my ejection fraction test.

I was nearly in tears with worry and anticipation.

I wanted so much for my readings to be in the normal range.

Thankfully there weren't many people waiting in the room with me, so I grabbed a magazine and my jacket to cover Frank, who was always ready to go to work for me. I let him pump for about ten minutes under there until my name was called.

As I laid on the examination table, my technician, a neat guy from Trinidad, began small talk. I wasn't in the mood. He had no idea how important this test was to me.

I sat up, looked directly in his eyes, and said, "This has to be normal. I need normal."

The technician replied in his cool Caribbean accent, "Well, if you believe it is normal, then it will be normal."

I could feel the cold, eerily-smooth gel lubrication and a wand rolling over my chest as I watched a live video of my heart pumping on the screen. I tried in vain to do an eyeball calculation of how wide my heart was expanding and contracting.

I couldn't help but notice how my heart looked so much like Frank and the way my heart was moving was so similar to how Frank moved.

Maybe I would be okay.

I didn't get instant results. My video would have to analyzed by a team.

I felt sick.

I didn't want to wait.

I wanted to know right at that moment.

Days went by. Two weeks went by.

I asked my rehab staff if they could look at my medical records to see if my test had come back.

They *were* back.

One staff member printed out the sheet with the new results.

What?

Oh my gosh!

Frank had done his job!

I would NOT need a defibrillator implant!

I spent a few minutes hugging the cardiac rehab staff and thanking them.

Then I went into the empty locker room and sobbed out many weeks' worth of pent-up worry.

I had never been more relieved.

I had never been this thankful.

I had never been this happy.

The Fittest I've Ever Been

As you know, heart patients are required to take periodic treadmill fitness tests called "stress tests." Patients are hooked up to a machine that records every major vital indicator (blood pressure, EKG, heart rate, and others) to see how the heart is behaving under pressure.

When I entered cardiac rehab, my stress test was predictable; I was extremely weak and far from fit. As I tried to run, it didn't take long before my calves cramped, and I hit the "stop" button to end the test.

My stress test was the sophisticated kind because it assessed "VO2 max," one of the most important fitness indicators. This required that I wear a mouthpiece as I ran to funnel my exhaled breath into a machine that measured the maximum capacity of my body's ability to transport and use oxygen during heavy exercise.

Predictably, my VO2 max was very low after my heart attack, but at the end of my rehab, my levels were higher than most of the fittest young exercise physiologist trainers in the rehab center! This meant that I had an advanced ability to intake oxygen and metabolize it throughout my body, when only just a few months earlier I could barely breathe. Wow!

In layman's terms, I had the "wind of a 20-year old college athlete." I had only just begun to improve.

And I had only just begun to run.

This has everything to do with hope.

(Or did it have to do with stem cells?)

Run, Jon Kyle, Run

The Columbus Marathon came around only two months after I started training outside and off the treadmill. I was up to an amazing 10 miles on my weekly long runs, but nowhere near the 18-22 that I needed to run a full marathon. So I decided to run my first half marathon (13.1 miles) instead of the full as was called for in my script.

But so what, right?

13.1 miles is a really long way for a recent heart attack victim. Heck, 13.1 miles is a long way for *anyone* to run! Laurie would be amazed, too, since a half marathon was my stated goal while in rehab.

I arrived at the starting area at around 7:15 a.m. for a 7:30 start. I had no idea that I was terribly late. I tried to push myself through the crowd but became stuck. There was no way I would be able to get to the area of slower runners in the back of the crowd. I couldn't make it to the only area where I would be allowed to enter onto the street.

Then someone shouted, "anyone who needs to can get in here! Come over here!"

A big area of the crowd rushed into a split in the barrier fence to the street just in time for the starting horn and fireworks.

Uh-oh!

I was in Corral 2 which was reserved only for seasoned runners, the second-fastest runners in the crowd. I thought, "Oh well, since I'm here I'll see if I can keep up."

Stupidly, I found myself flying down the street but being passed by absolutely everyone! I raced to Mile 1 as dozens—*hundreds* of runners—smoked me. Then Mile 2. Past Mile 4! 5! Because so many runners passed me it seemed as though I was running in slow motion when, in fact, my legs were carrying me faster than I ever knew I could run.

I was wearing a heart monitor belt and watch that the rehab staff recommended. I could see that my heart rate was getting high. I blew it. I should have known better because I read many articles about getting caught up in the moment and starting out too fast. Any runner knows this is the absolute worst thing that a runner can do in long races. I was running at my maximum capacity among veteran racers who were taking it easy for the first few miles! How dumb! *A rookie mistake indeed!*

According to my split time, I ran a 58-minute 10K (lightning fast for me!). Then I hit Mile 7. This is where volunteers were handing out energy gels. I thought, "Hmmm." Energy gels would give me the energy I needed after starting out too fast.

I took two gel packets and sucked them both down. The contents were gooey and tasted like delicious cake-icing. Not too long after I swallowed the last bit from the second package, I was in serious trouble.

"Boom-boom-BOOM-*BOOM*!" My heart was beating out of my chest. I had never felt more jittery and I was panicking. I had to stop running and calm myself down.

Oh no, *not again!* Not *now!* Not during my first half-marathon! *Could this be another heart attack?* I decided to sit down on the pavement behind the cheering crowd.

"Wait a minute," I thought. "What was in that gel energy stuff?"

I raised myself upright and picked a discarded gel container off the ground and realized that it was packed with caffeine. I didn't use caffeine, so I immediately knew that I was simply having a normal reaction to a drug that was foreign to my body.

Now I had *really* blown it. I was walking. Where was this in my script? I had to walk to see if my caffeinated jitters would subside for me to feel okay enough to start running again.

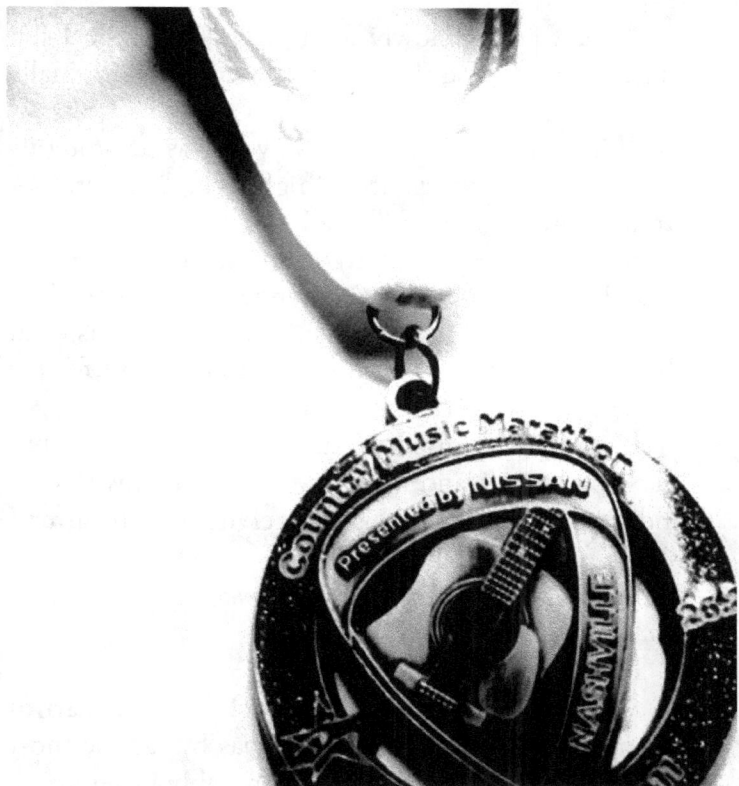

"My First Marathon Medal"

It's like Olympic gold to me. I am alive.
I am outlandish! (Many more to come.)

After walking slowly for nearly a full mile I felt much better and settled into the pace I had originally trained for.

This was more like it! Now I was thoroughly enjoying the experience, "high-fiving" spectators, smiling and clapping for all the bands who were graciously playing at many locations along the way, thanking the volunteers who handed me water or Gatorade, and absorbing the positive energy. This is what the race experience was supposed to be about for me in the first place. (Lesson learned!)

I completed my half marathon in a slow but respectable 2:19, and I finished the last half with ease and grace. And I did this only eight months after I nearly died!

I completed a big race only eight months after contemplating suicide!

I was so proud of myself.

And I realized that slow is fine! The slow part of the marathon (the second half) was by far the most enjoyable part of the race. I am probably never going to win a race, but I can participate and truly enjoy races.

So instead of letting myself die or become incapacitated I can now say that I ran a half marathon!

Please know that I'm not trying to toot my own horn. I'm merely thrilled that I wrote a script for myself and my mind made it a reality (even though the script was for the full marathon).

The detail of that script was powerful. For instance, of course I *had* to wear black shorts, and fortunately I owned a pair. But I had to go out and find a lime green tank top even though the morning of race day was a 38-degree start in mid-October in Ohio, but I absolutely insisted on wearing my green tank top. After all it was in the script. That explains why I missed the sweat drip, drip, dripping off my shimmering skin. It wasn't really hot enough for my skin to shimmer or to spread my DNA. Still, the experience was wonderful and will always be one of my greatest accomplishments.

Six months later I ran another half marathon, (The Capital City Half Marathon, also in Columbus) and I finished in 2:25 (very slow), but this time, because I was paranoid about the mistakes I made in my debut half marathon, I simply enjoyed being alive and able to run. It was magical.

That same spring, I attempted my first full marathon, The Country Music Marathon in Nashville (26.2 miles!).

By any competitive marathoner's standards, my first marathon turned out to be a disaster. I finished in 5:52. 70-year-olds were having their way with me. I wasn't trained for the steep hills that zapped me early on and nearly put me on the ground in the last few miles. *But I did it.*

I ran slowly to Mile 18. (Wow!) And then I hit "the wall" and basically crawled the last eight miles. I could have been dead. But I participated in a marathon and finished it. *Awesome!* I will always be proud of this time because I was thrilled to be alive.

At about Mile 19, I was with a pack of runners -turned-walkers and our legs felt like lead. I was probably not breaking 2.5 miles per hour. A young man in my pack looked at me and said, "Do you think we should start running now?"

I said, "Go ahead. Good luck. I'll see you later at the finish line."

The young man started running in slow motion as my group of very slow walkers blew past him at our snail's pace! We all cracked up, laughing so hard that some of us had to stop walking for a few seconds to regroup. Then a beer stop appeared.

A local company was handing out beer, supposedly good for replenishing carbs near the end of a marathon.

My group of turtles all grabbed a cup of beer.

I said, "To life!"

"To life!" The entire group replied.

They had no idea how much that toast meant to me. And even though I was in agony, this beer was the most delicious beer I had ever drunk. That particular moment was the most memorable part of the marathon.

We separated over the last three miles. I kept on trudging along even when my leg muscles screamed as they confronted one more big hill before the last slide in.

I dug deep down and ran the last .2 of the 26.2 miles and crossed the finish line with dignity. I didn't finish anywhere close to last, which was a victory.

I completed a marathon!

Since then I have run the full Columbus Marathon (in 5:14: I'm getting a bit faster) and I have signed up for another Nashville. I hope to get down to 4:30 someday. So as you can tell, mine is not a story about nearly dying and placing in the Boston Marathon or beating 20-year-olds. That would not be realistic for someone who never ran before and is not likely realistic for you either. I'm talking about pure symbolism and accomplishment through attempting outlandish things such as simply *finishing* marathons. I finish slow, but I'm much faster than dead people.

OUTLANDISH!

I could be dead but I am alive. I have an abundance of hope. I am magnificent.

As I mature in my athletic endeavors, I foresee diversifying from marathons and declaring "I'm a cyclist," or "I'm a swimmer—a rower"—a triathlete—or anything I choose to do as long as I continue to be magnificently active—*because I can.* You can too.

My Artery-Scrubbing Diet

By now you know that either stem cells, self-designed biofeedback (my heart puppets), and/or intense exercise (or a combination of these) allowed me to thrive after my heart attack. I have neglected to this point to mention that perhaps the biggest lifestyle change I made after my heart attack was becoming a vegan.

This is amazing because I have had a lifelong love affair with meat.

In fact, I was on the low (or no) carb and "eat-all-the meat-you-want" diet for more years than I want to think about.

When I was in my twenties and thirties, a typical day of meals would be something like this:

Breakfast: 6 scrambled eggs smothered in cheddar cheese and fried in real butter. (I would even eat a hunk of butter while watching the eggs cook.) I'd wash the eggs down with a huge glass of whole milk and maybe top the meal off with an entire package of sausage.

Lunch: A triple cheeseburger with bacon and mayo or three or four pieces of cube steak that I fried myself in olive oil because olive oil is "good for me." To add balance, I'd include a big bowl of broccoli smothered in butter.

Dinner: A huge steak with salad and thick, three-cheese dressing with half a package of homemade bacon and Parmesan cheese blanketing the contents.

Eating like this is insane.

With my family history of early heart disease, there is very little wonder why I had a heart attack.

Very soon after the heart attack, I did a lot of research about food that help heart attack survivors stay alive longer. I am convinced that eating a zero-meat, zero-dairy, zero-oil diet (three of my very favorite things to eat) is the way to go. There are good books out there showing evidence that eating like this can reverse heart disease (unplug clogged arteries).

So ever since my heart attack I have refrained from eating meat or dairy, and I have limited my oil to an occasional spray or drip to keep food from sticking.

I spend a lot of time creating new recipes. Now my typical day of eating consists of (for example):

Breakfast: A bowl of whole grain cereal with no added sugar or salt with a cup or two of almond milk.

Lunch: A salad (only veggies and no cheese) topped with balsamic vinegar (Not a vinaigrette! Just vinegar.) or a bowl of lentils garnished with chopped raw cabbage.

Dinner: Pinto beans and brown rice sprinkled with hot pepper flakes and zero-fat corn bread that I made myself with almond milk. (This one is, by far, my favorite!)

At first this diet was horrifying. I constantly craved meat and I experienced severe withdrawal pangs. For instance, at my grocery store there is a "hot bar" with fried food. Every time I shopped I was lured to the forbidden fried chicken fingers that were irresistible to me before the heart attack. I would put my head near the hot chicken fingers and sniff as hard and strong as I could, my mouth watering to overflowing.

I would also dream of steak dripping with blood and mashed potatoes slathered with butter.

But thinking about how I would be able to keep living and also reverse my heart disease kept me on track, completely abstaining from any meat, dairy, or oil.

After a few months, my lipids doctor said that he didn't think it would be a bad idea if I ate fish, and in particular, trout.

I did add some fish to my diet for a short time, but it started to taste like grease. The smell of fish flesh made me nauseous. Yuck! It is hard for me, once one of the world's unabashed carnivores, to realize that I had completely lost my taste for animal products of any kind.

But I feel a lot better. And I will keep this up for the rest of my life. Just like anything else, it's not hard after you get used to it.

I know how hard it is to do, but you should seriously consider becoming an oil-free vegan too.

I am convinced that it's another path to creating a "bionic heart."

My Heart Regenerated Itself

In my stem cell trial appointments I had to get periodic MRI tests to see if my heart was healing. My original MRI test showed some damaged tissue.

Remember, stem cells are supposed to HEAL hearts by repairing the tissue and promoting blood vessel growth.

From the time of my tragedy to my 18-month post-heart attack checkup, I had been running like a madman. I logged 40 to 50 miles every week and had run many races: four 5Ks (I ran one 5K in just under 27:00 which was thrilling to me), a 5-mile Thanksgiving "Turkey Trot (46:15 and I'll take it)," two half marathons and a full marathon. I was sure my heart had to be somehow improving. But it was better than that.

My cardiologist informed me that my MRI tests showed no damage.

NONE.

Zero!

Nada!

And my EKG test was 100% normal. I am a freak of nature.

I asked him to repeat what he said. I needed to hear it again. I needed to savor it.

"You have no damage," he repeated.

"Stem cells?" I asked.

My doctor shook his head, "I just don't know."

So did the stem cells repair my heart or was it my positive thinking and will to become healthy again—to become an athlete—to become a runner—a marathoner, that made miracles happen?

Funny, when I was sad and suicidal, I wanted nothing more than to know I had the stem cells. Now that I am healed and healthy again, I want to believe that my will to be healthy is what healed my heart.

Besides, everyone has stem cells in their bodies.

Maybe I called mine up?

Maybe my strict vegan diet was the reason I was healthy again?

Or could it be all of these things?

I could have given up on myself. Today I'm thriving. Now it's time for you to start on your path to a thriving life.

Don't Give Up Hope

You are probably in a state of despair.

I was there too not so long ago. I understand what you are going through.

Perhaps you're finding out that only people who have actually suffered through the experience of a personal health tragedy can possibly know how you feel or truly know what you need right now.

I've been there.

Just try to understand that although things seem cold and dark for you at this moment, you have the power to make yourself better just like I did.

The Formula for Your Recovery

Hope. The formula for your recovery is simply hope.

Right now, you need a lot of it.

Believe me, I know.

We both know that things couldn't be more serious for you.

Emergency sirens are blaring all around you.

You have to harvest every bit of hope that exists inside you and in the world, and you have to do this right now.

It's time to call up your reserves of strength and hope.

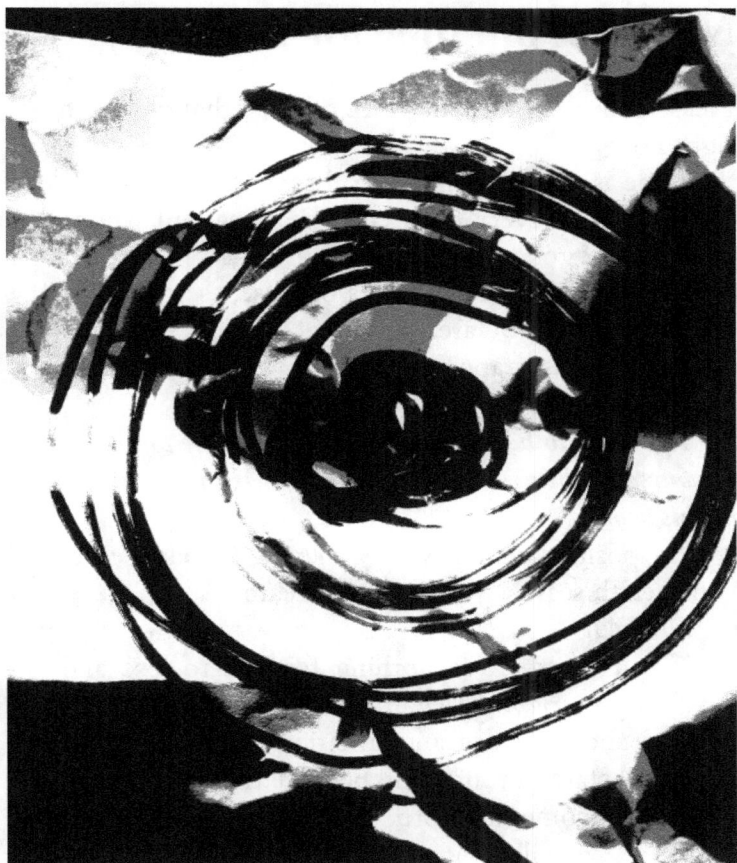

"Hope"

This is my abstract target with dark spaces on the edges representing potentially dangerous outcomes. Hope is a target you must hit.

My Voice of Hope for You

Please consider mine the voice of hope that you need right now.

Mine is the missing voice that should be speaking directly to every frightened heart patient who is yearning for good news.

I know your circumstances because, as you know, I've been where you are.

You need assurance.

You may not get it.

You have to be brave enough to continue to give it to yourself when no one else will. This is the big lesson of this book.

I'm positive that having a *better life* than before your health scare is your wildest dream.

Dream it!

If you do, there is nothing for you to lose and absolutely *everything* to gain.

Very shortly your transformation will begin.

It will start in your mind because that is where all positive outcomes are born.

Then you'll witness your metamorphosis from hopeless and sick to your new, magnificent physical self.

I want you to look back on what you're going through and consider your experience a gift. (Ugh! *I know!* You're cringing but you should be open to the possibility that your awful illness is actually a blessing. It's an opportunity to learn and grow, as in "What doesn't kill you makes you stronger.")

For those of you who are saying, "I'm too far gone," or "I don't want to give myself false hope," please remember this simple truth:

Without hope you join the walking dead until you die.

In other words, you either find hope or you might as well be dead.

And if you don't find hope, you will be dead soon enough.

(This is harsh, but it's simply true.)

You are not ready to die yet.

A Special Message for Hospitalized Readers

If you're in a hospital bed suffering through the lowest point of what is by far the most upsetting experience of your life, I'm so sorry.

It seems as if you're merely along for the ride. I know how scary that feeling is.

More than just about any other time during my medical situation, I needed a strong voice of hope when I was laid up fighting for my life.

But don't worry.

Now that you are reading this book, you have a positive voice to steer you through the darkness, and you will get through this.

I know that your mind is going crazy.

Perhaps you feel tied down because you are attached to wires and beeping machines with annoying flashing lights.

Maybe you are flat out incapacitated. Whatever you are going through, there is nothing pleasant about it.

I want to tell you something:

I love you.

Did your eyebrows go up?

Yes, I know that we've never met and I'm telling you that I love you. That might seem a bit strange.

Saying "I love you" is a cherished, often private phrase that is normally reserved for the people closest to us.

But if you think about it, few experiences bond strangers tighter than life-changing experiences they share in common.

I had a heart attack and that changed my world forever.

The heart condition that overtook your life will change your world forever too.

That's why I know you, and just like soldiers in war, we are fighters in the same battle—staying alive.

We made it through the horrifying experience of surviving our diseases to this point.

We're brothers and sisters at heart.

So of course I care about and love you.

I know that you need all the love that you can get at this moment.

I *know* you!

Now I'm going to open up to you about something very personal…

When I was in the hospital during and immediately after my heart attack, I quietly cried the whole time with tears continuously streaming down my face.

I couldn't help it.

Even when I wasn't outwardly crying, inside I was weeping.

I was sad because I had lost my good health which I had previously taken for granted and because I was so scared about what might be coming next.

Was there something else lurking?

A stroke?

Another heart attack that would "take care of the unfinished job?"

Would I be able to exercise again?

Would other body parts fail me?

Everything seemed imminently bleak and terribly frightening.

Most of all, I was sad because, no matter what, I would now and forevermore be known as a "heart patient."

I never took any medications and now—BOOM—now I was required to swallow a daily heart cocktail tonic of different colored pills of all sizes—*and for the rest of my life?*

Now I would have to explain the enormous blemish on my record to potential employers with my shameful preexisting health condition. I felt like damaged goods. I was a shell of the previous self who existed only a few hours before; I was in deep mourning for him.

Dealing with all these dire circumstances at once, I cried, which seems entirely appropriate.

If you're in the hospital reading this, I know you must be experiencing similar feelings, and you are surely very sad, too.

The stench of hospital sterility that you have to smell right now is still in my nose today. And I will never, ever eat Jello or a popsicle or drink apple juice again! I know you know what I mean.

So if you need to cry right now please go ahead. It's okay. I cried so much in the hospital that my medical records say (literally), "The patient was teary-eyed and obviously very sad." Well, duh! What is the expected behavior for a new heart patient? Maybe my doctors expected me to smile and be thrilled that I almost died and that my life would be forever changed, so they could write, "The patient was smiling from ear to ear and obviously in bliss"?

I've been crying for you while writing this section. That's right—tears have been flowing and my throat is just about closed up. Thinking about you brings me back to those dark, hopeless feelings I endured, and, because my feelings are genuine, I weep tears of hardcore empathy for you.

Knowing that you and untold thousands of people are currently feeling as dark and hopeless as I did back then is hard for me to take, and nothing—absolutely *nothing*—is worse than being stuck in hopelessness.

I don't want you to lose hope. This is precisely what this book is for and why I am glad that a copy came to you in time for you to use it.

Soon you'll be drinking in a big glass of delicious, nourishing, powerful hope.

Hug Yourself

You know, if I saw you I'd hug you, so I could transfer my excess reserves of overflowing hope into you.

Nobody did that for me. Hugging isn't in very many job descriptions. Maybe more doctors would feel an impulse to hug if they came to understand the injustice of having their body reject the very organ that sustains life.

But let's be real—medical professionals are there to treat you, not hug.

I want to be clear; I am not knocking medical professionals. I love my cardiologist, my lipids doctor, and my general healthcare physician. Doctors are great because they save lives, and they do an excellent job of practicing medicine. They try their hardest to keep their patients alive. I personally thanked many of them for not letting me die. But I couldn't rely on them to give me the kind of hope I needed. I still can't.

Most doctors would probably agree that they can't completely understand all of their patients' emotional needs. They would if they could. But with the stress they endure, the number of patients they need to see, and only so many hours in a day, they simply don't have time. Who can blame them?

Nurses don't usually have time to hug either, but they are angels. They work extremely hard. Most are very kind and have tender hearts. But like doctors, they can't possibly know how to reach inside our souls that are so desperate for emotional nourishment. They can't give you the light of hope in your darkest moments of fear and despair. Nurses will never have the kind of time needed to cultivate deep relationships and listen to all of our personal stories, wishes, hopes, and dreams.

Hospital chaplains and social workers have more time to hug. They offer comfort, and they listen. But they're never going to be your get-well coaches. There are too many other sick people they have to see today.

Your friends and family members will be glad to hug you. They love and support you because they can't imagine life without you. They can encourage you, but they have their own lives. They can't get inside your skin no matter how hard they try, and they don't know what you need most; that's up to you. *That's inside of you.*

Right now, you need to know that you are going to feel, look, and be physically magnificent in good time. That's a lot to ask and might seem impossible. Perhaps this is why nobody can commit to giving you the continuous high level of positive encouragement

and reinforcement you will need to achieve high ex-
pectation health goals.

Only you can do this.

You have to be willing to write a new script
featuring an inspirational story about your
amazing recovery.

Your doctors won't. Your family can't.

If you believe in God, then he can help.

*But YOU have to robustly cultivate constant,
growing hope that will bring you into physical magnificence, and you must do this with the highest levels of
passion and vigor.*

In other words, you have to learn to hug yourself.

You must recognize this right now if you want to
get better. It's up to you.

Your Rebirth Begins Now

If you are alive right now and you can read this and
you are breathing, you can have hope.

You need hope for your rebirth.

You need hope to plan your full recovery and have
no expectations for anything less.

Hope gives you the will to live and refuse to die.

But most of all, you must tell yourself—you must
believe—that you will thrive and become an inspi-

ration to everyone in your life and even become an inspiration to yourself.

So begin right now; tell yourself that you have the power inside to make a full recovery and that you will indeed be better than you ever were before. Tell yourself that nothing will stop you from becoming a physical phenomenon and that you will feel fantastic soon.

Now, look at your face in the mirror and say,

"I am going to kick my heart disease's ass."

Then go do it.

I want you to cling to this book, so you'll have access to my voice of hope whenever you need a refill.

Your future doesn't have to be bleak now that you have an empathetic voice on your side.

I'm happy now because I know you feel hope.

Declare Your Athleticism

Everyone who experiences a heart attack must decide: have your ass kicked by your heart disease or decide to kick your heart disease's ass.

Make the right decision by getting your blood pumping with physical activity because all diseases respond to movement and physical exercise.

This involves becoming an athlete.

Don't let this sound intimidating.

The definition of "athlete" is simply a regular participant in a sport.

So no matter what condition you are in right now—stuck in a hospital, can't currently walk, can't breathe well, can't whatever, say this out loud:

I am an athlete.

Now Choose Your Way to Move

It's up to you to determine what you will do to achieve your goal. It should be an activity that you enjoy and that will keep you from allowing your body to deteriorate. You must do something to wake up your physical spirit and heal yourself.

Get more specific by establishing a physical activity goal and choose your sport.

I hope you choose running, but you can go for rock climbing, ice skating, power-walking, or whatever else inspires you to help your heart and turn your life around.

Be Outlandish

If you want to thrive you must be outlandish. If you choose running, being outlandish is very easy. You are already familiar with my goal to become a marathoner.

If you are a mountain climber, you will climb a tall mountain, maybe Mt. Everest, but you'll start with a flight of stairs and then proceed to a small hill.

Climbing a small hill is an amazing accomplishment for someone who might otherwise be dead. Someday you'll climb a big hill. That will be even more amazing. You will work your way up to Mt. Everest.

If you choose walking as your sport, maybe your outlandish goal is walking 100 miles. Maybe it's walking across an entire state or a continent. Meanwhile, walking that 50-foot "lap" across the hospital floor or up your street and back may be the first accomplishment needed to achieve your outlandish goal.

Choose your outlandish goal for your sport right now.

Write Your Script

You must write your own script. It's your story for your bright future. Please remember that it has to be vivid and detailed enough for you to be perpetually inspired when you dream and when you exercise.

It's your movie.

Make it thrilling and inspirational.

Dress the Part

Heart disease is very tricky. You can't let it trick you any further. Why not trick it instead?

You'll do this by realizing that right now you are at a very important crossroads and many of your successes and failures are in your mind. They are stories that you tell yourself. You have to fix your mind right now so you too can become bionic.

You may have heard the phrase "Dress for your next job." This describes ambitious people, say, a teller at a bank who wants to be the bank president. It's similar for you and your outlandish health goal; you have to dress for the part of your future physical magnificence.

Just like dressing for the next job you have to dress for the athlete you aspire to be. This is one of the best ways to trick your mind into buying into your new self because if it sees you looking like a tennis pro, you could become a damn good tennis player. So go out and get clothes and gear that match your new physical fitness goals.

When I decided that I was going to become a runner, I got into the running shoe research mania: What kind of arches did I have? (Answer: Flat to normal.) How do I pronate? (I overpronate fairly severely with frequent heel strikes.)

Proudly, I ended up splurging on three pairs of very expensive running shoes, and I am happy to report that I just bought a fourth pair that is waiting in a box to be opened a month before my next marathon.

Even with the expensive shoes, I have four black toenails, and two out of the four are on my big toes. That's how much I run! Many runners have them, and I consider my black toenails to be my war scars and my badges of honor.

I can spend hours at sporting goods stores going rack by rack to continue building my running wardrobe. I don't remember when I have ever had so much fun!

Currently I have at least 10 pairs of running shorts. (I like the short-shorts with the leg splits because I look more like a fast runner even though I hate to admit that I am slow as a slug.) I also have plenty of good running socks; and I spared no expense to avoid blisters. (The best socks seem to come from South Africa for some reason.)

And along with my prized green tank, I have an array of winter and summer technical shirts that get heavy use. I'm also collecting the race shirts that are given out in the goody bags. They are beginning to pile up.

When I'm in my running costume I love to get a "runners nod" from other runners. This gesture means, "I know you. I am a runner too. Godspeed." It's thrilling because I AM A RUNNER. I should be dead! And when I run in marathons, I look like a marathoner because *I AM A MARATHONER.*

Whatever your sport, look the part to play the part. And more importantly, your mind will acknowledge your look, and then your body will follow by making you become the athlete you are dressing to become.

Create Your Version of "Frank"

Figure out how to visualize your heart improving and even healing.

You know how I do it.

How will you?

Don't Eat Meat or Dairy

Just don't. You'll be glad.

Expect a Medical Miracle

We don't know what medical science will reveal tomorrow, next month, or next year. Maybe stem cells or something better will be available in your not-so-distant future. Hold on to the hope that medical research will provide healing possibilities for your heart. Tomorrow might be the day a "nurse angel" tells you that they have something new that you will want to know more about. Until then, take care of yourself and prepare for your medical miracle.

Your Future in a Nutshell

What you are going through now is just a temporary setback. The road to your recovery is a choice you have to make right now. Think about the magnificent renewal that can start now if you let it.

Who cares what the tests say?

It doesn't really matter what your doctors say.

It matters what you believe.

Adjust your attitude and get ready for (literally) the fight of your life.

You will beat this. Period.

There can be no excuses. Not only will you survive, you will thrive. Now it is time.

Now Go Become Bionic

It's such a great feeling to have a formula of hope, isn't it? Take it and make it happen for you.

I named this book "Becoming Bionic" because the definition for the word 'bionic' is having superhuman strength or capacity.

I call my heart "My Bionic Heart."

It's strong.

It's superhuman.

Why not?

And why not imagine that you also have a bionic heart?

Tell your mind to turn your body into something much different than it is right now.

Let your mind transform your body into the physically magnificent body it deserves to be.

I don't care how old you are, what your circumstances are, or your current health status. I made it through and you will, too.

Good luck!

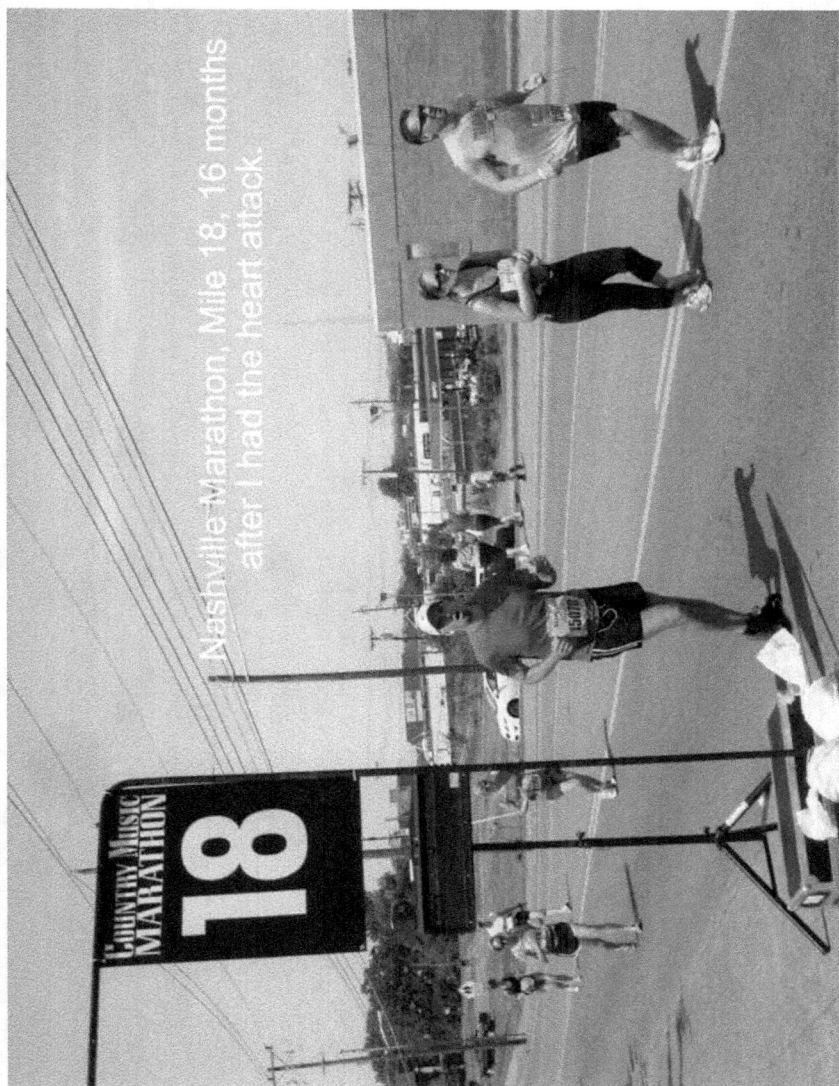

Nashville Marathon, Mile 18, 16 months after I had the heart attack.

Start now.

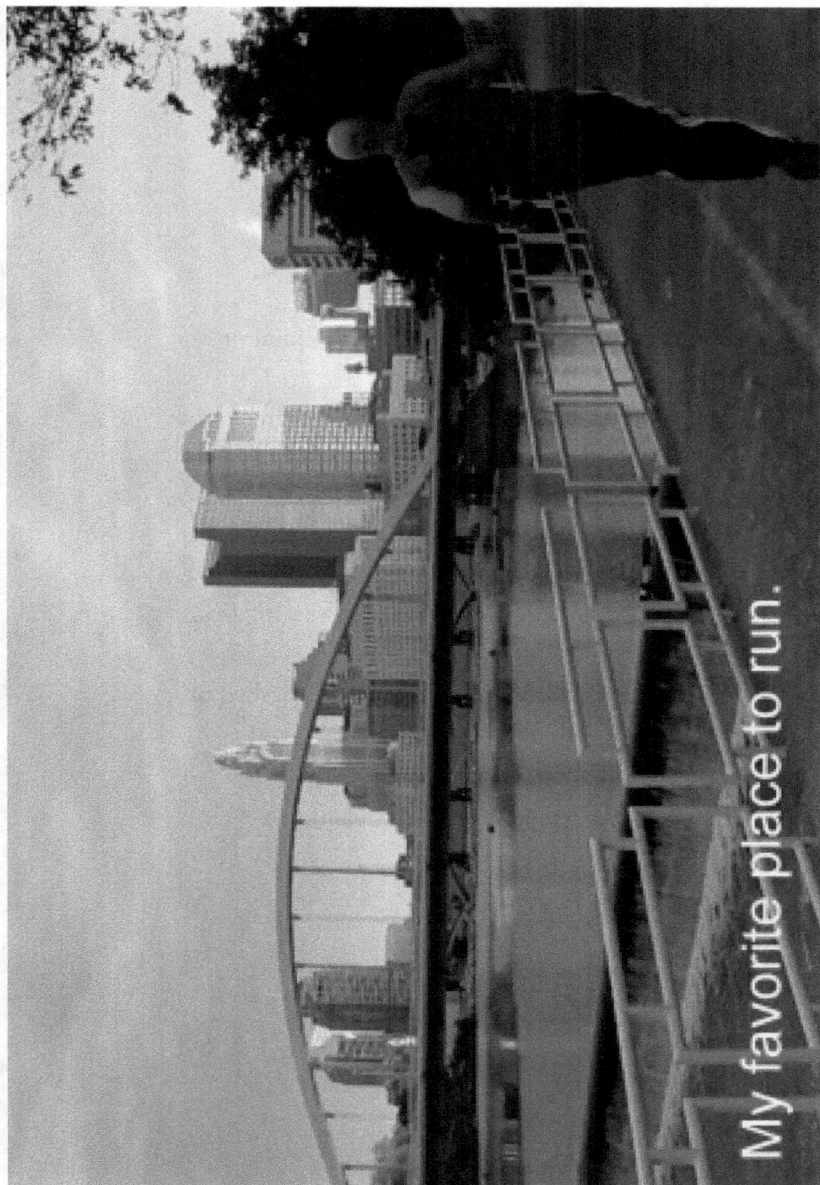

My favorite place to run.

My Prayer for Dying

Lord, don't let me die in a hospital or on a couch.

Please take me as I race down a greenway trail or up a city street with my running costume drenched in sweat.

And I'll leave this Earth magnificent, outlandish, and unafraid,

With pure joy and happiness ringing from my last gasps,

And if I'm found with my face smashed on hard, cold pavement,

I will cheer from heaven,

"Sweet, dignity! Sweet, sweet dignity!"

Amen.

My Goal

Richard Simmons is my hero. He amazes me.
In much the same way he reaches obese people who are desperate to be thin and healthy, I want to reach heart attack victims who need help getting better. I want to run around the world and meet millions of people just like Richard does. I want to do this because I sincerely care. When something like a near-fatal heart attack alters your life, priorities shift. Dumb things don't matter anymore and most things are dumb. But helping people is not dumb. I know people need my help because *I needed my help!* As a person who truly knows what it's like to face mortality brought forth by a heart malfunction, I want to be there for others. I want to run marathons with others I've inspired. We can wear tee-shirts that say "I had a heart attack—what's your excuse?" We can cry together as we rejoice at the finish line. There is a voice inside that is clearly telling me that this is what I must do. Just like Richard Simmons does for obese people.

Thanks to the Ross Heart Hospital at
The Ohio State University Medical Center
"I'm' so glad I had a heart attack in Columbus, Ohio!"

My kick-butt cardiologist, Dr. Vincent Pompili, MD
My incredible lipids doctor, Scott H. Merryman, MD
and my caring General Practitioner, John McConaghy, MD

Meet other bionic men and women on
becomingbionic.com

We will encourage each other
into physical magnificence.

www.ingramcontent.com/pod-product-compliance
Lightning Source LLC
Chambersburg PA
CBHW050540280326
41933CB00011B/1667